Meal Planning

Meal Planning For Weight Loss

By

Bring On Fitness

information contained within this document, including, but not limited to, errors, omissions, or inaccuracies.

About Bring On Fitness

Our passion for fitness gave life to **Bring On Fitness**. We started with the goal of helping as many people as we can. To educate, motivate and to help change peoples lives for the better. Bring On Fitness is not only for the fitness enthusiasts, but also for the beginner. We strongly believe nothing is more important than learning the basics and creating a strong foundation in both nutrition - through meal planning, and in exercise - by following a specific plan. This is just as important for the beginner, as it is for the experienced athlete.

We set high standards for ourselves, the information we share, and the products we carry. Our goal is to provide you with exceptional products that suit your needs and the knowledge and motivation to help you work towards and achieve your health and fitness goals.

Check us out at www.bringonfitness.com

"Our Mission is to have a positive impact in changing peoples lives. We will deliver the best possible fitness and nutrition solutions that will empower people to achieve their health and fitness goals."

Table of Contents

Introduction

Do you want to lose weight? Do you want to eat more healthily? Do you want your meals to be more varied and interesting? Great, then meal planning for weight loss is for you!

This guide will teach you:

- How to save money by buying only the food you need
- How to take all the guesswork out of your meals
- How to save yourself time by preparing meals in advance
- How to change bad eating habits for good ones
- How to get more variety into your meals
- How to achieve better nutritional balance
- What ratio of carbs, fats, and proteins you should be eating
- What the different food groups do for your body
- And of course, HOW to meal plan for weight loss

Are you ready? Then let's get started!

Chapter 1

Why Meal Plan?

The benefits of meal planning are great and can help you in a variety of ways:

1. **Save Money, Buy Only What You Need**

All of us like to save money where we can. Food is one of the areas where overspending can be quite excessive. When you don't plan meals in advance, going shopping can be just like taking the kids to the toy store and telling them they can have whatever they want. It's just too easy to walk up and down the aisles while picking up whatever suits your fancy.

If you're feeling stressed, hormonal, tired, or hungry, you will be craving sweet treats and high-carb foods, which make you feel better for a short time. However, you'll soon be back to feeling stressed, hormonal, tired, and hungry all over again.

Not only is this random buying bad for your bank balance, but it also wreaks havoc on your waistline!

When you sit down and make a meal plan, shopping becomes simple. You're able to make a specific list of all the items you need. Thus, when you're in the shop, the random picking of what you fancy is gone. Instead, you know exactly what's required. Now, it just takes a bit of self-discipline to not pick up "want" items along the way. A want item is one that you want but don't need. Don't give in to wants; stick only to your needs.

2. **Take all the Guesswork out of Meals**

By making a weekly or monthly meal plan, you always know exactly what's for breakfast, lunch, and dinner each day. This is beneficial in two ways. First, you don't spend all day thinking about food, wondering what you're going to eat. This kind of thinking makes you hungry and leads you to make bad choices and even binge on food you know you shouldn't eat. Meal planning takes the stress out of always wondering what to make. Food can become really boring when you always leave the decisions to the last minute. This is because you become inclined to choose something quick and easy that you eat too often. This type of food tends to fail you on several fronts; it is typically of low nutritional value, often carb heavy, and boring as hell to eat.

Our lives are hectic; it isn't wrong that we want to make it easy. Rather than making the same boring food day in day out or just giving up altogether and ordering takeout (expensive and high calorie), meal planning can help you make things better by making better choices.

3. **Save Time, Prepare Ahead**

This is one of the most advantageous parts of meal planning. If you know you won't have time to cook a meal from fresh on Tuesday night (because you go to that class you enjoy, or whatever), no problem! You can make that evening meal in advance and freeze it, or make it the evening before and keep it in the fridge.

Meal planning lets you think ahead. Be sure to look at your meal plan alongside your weekly schedule so you know well in advance if you're going to need to be pro-active and make something ahead of time. The idea is to reduce your food stress, not make it worse by making you have too much to do when your time is already limited.

Get organized, and make as much as you can ahead of time. It would make you feel so great, knowing that everything is organized and ready to go.

4. Change Bad Eating Habits to Good Ones

Just like when you're in the store, shopping with no plan, it's really easy to get into bad habits at home, too. Eating junk between meals, especially on your day off when you have time on your hands, can be a big problem. By meal planning, you can alleviate this in two ways. First, the junk food won't be in your kitchen cupboards to tempt you. Second, you can make better choices for yourself about the snacks you can eat. You can even build them into your meal plan.

Cravings can be deadly when trying to lose weight. Many people are tempted to reduce their food intake too quickly, or start skipping meals, which leaves them feeling hungry. When you're hungry, you crave food, and I'm not talking carrot sticks and celery, but chocolate, chips, bread, and sweet treats. This can lead to ignoring rational thoughts and listening instead to the ones telling you that it's only one piece of chocolate, it's only one slice of pizza, and it's only one bag of chips. Before you know it, you've eaten enough calories to sustain yourself for an entire week in just a few hours. Use the meal plans to help you reduce your calorie intake gradually. This doesn't mean you have to eat a whole lot less; it just means you exchange the bad foods for good ones.

Use meal planning to build in treats you can have and enjoy without remorse. This will build on good eating habits and help to break the bad. Remember, the more you deny yourself food, the hungrier you will become.

5. Get More Variety into your Meals

The problem with just winging it and not making any plans about what you're going to eat is that meals often totally lack variety. This means you eat the same stuff again and again, week in week out. It's boring, but more importantly, it's nutritionally a disaster. You need variety in your diet, a good range of healthy vegetables, and a balance of protein, fat, carbohydrate, etc. Otherwise, your body would lack the nutrients needed to be healthy. This doesn't only have a big effect on your waistline; it can also be very detrimental to your health, making you prone to illness and disease, both mental and physical.

6. Create a Better Nutritional Balance

Variety really is linked to balance. You will have heard the phrase, "Eat a balanced diet," many times, but what does it actually mean?

You will have heard of proteins, carbohydrates, fiber, fats (sometimes called lipids), and of course, water. These are all known as "macronutrients," which essentially means you need a lot of them for survival. Then, you also need "micronutrients," which means you don't need a whole lot, but they are essential in small amounts. These are vitamins and minerals.

Together, these play essential roles within your body:
- Energy production
- Growth and repair
- Maintaining a healthy metabolic function

When trying to lose weight, different people have different needs. It depends on the lifestyle you lead – sedentary or active. It depends on your gender, age, weight, and build. It may take a bit of tweaking to find the right balance for you. As a guide, a balanced meal should be divided in this way:

One Quarter Carbohydrate (energy food). This includes foods, such as potatoes, rice, bread, pasta, couscous, quinoa, oats, barley, and other cereals. Wholegrain carbohydrates that have not been stripped of all their beneficial fiber are digested a lot more slowly in the body and provide a gradual energy release. They also make you feel full and can thus help prevent snacking between meals.

Highly processed carbohydrates, such as white bread, white rice, white flour, and so on, are converted very quickly into glucose. This produces excess in your body and can wreak havoc on your metabolism. Try to avoid all processed carbohydrates whenever possible.

One Quarter Protein (growth and repair). This includes meat, fish, eggs, dairy products, nuts, and seeds.

One Quarter Vegetables and One Eighth Fruit (metabolic function). Try to go for the best mix of color you can in order to achieve the best range of nutrients. Dark green leafy vegetables, such as kale, watercress, and spinach, are king when it comes to providing a broad range of micronutrients, as well as fiber. Red vegetables, such as beets, red cabbage, tomatoes, and bell peppers, are full of antioxidants.

One Sixteenth Dairy. The jury is really out on dairy products at the moment. On the one hand, people say it is un-natural for us to consume dairy products. On the other hand, dairy products do contain a lot of beneficial micronutrients. If you include dairy, try to use organic goat milk instead of cows' milk. Buy organic, grass- fed products.

One Sixteenth Treats. If you need to have treats, then build it into your daily ratio – up to one sixteenth of your daily ratio, but no more. It would be better to add this allowance to your fruit and veg ratio if you can manage it.

Whenever possible, eat raw vegetables and fruit, as cooking will destroy some of the nutritional value. Buy organic products that are locally grown as much as you can. Intensive farming has stripped the earth of many micronutrients, depriving us of important minerals. This means that even though we are eating foods that should give us a good nutritional balance in micronutrients, we still won't be getting enough. Pesticides and herbicides are not good for our health, and even if you wash your veg, you can't remove what the vegetable has absorbed while growing. This is why buying organic or growing your own is better.

Chapter 2

Foods in Focus

So now you know why meal planning is so great. You understand how it can help you in your quest to lose weight by helping you avoid buying your *wants* rather than *needs*. You have a guide to the ratio of foods you should be consuming to help you choose foods from each group. Now, it's time to look at what those foods provide you, so you can make the best choices when meal planning.

You don't have to be a food scientist to plan balanced meals to promote weight loss, but understanding foods better can help. There are plenty of resources available on the internet that can do all the work out for you. Just search "meal plans for weight loss."

Fat

Fat is probably the most misunderstood substance we consume when it comes to dieting. Let's get one thing totally straight: fat is an ESSENTIAL part of our diet.

Fat is your body's back up energy source. When you have used all available glucose, the primary energy source, for your energy requirements, your body will start using fat from your fat cells for energy.

Some vitamins, such as A, D, E, and K, are only soluble in fat. This means that without fat, you couldn't use these vitamins in your body.

It's also necessary to produce essential fatty acids that promote brain development, help control inflammation, and assist in blood clotting. They also keep your skin (the largest organ of your body) and hair healthy.

Fats have a higher calorific value (9 per gram) than either carbohydrates or protein (both 4 per gram).

Not all fats are made equal. You may well have heard of saturated or unsaturated fats. This lets you know what type of fatty acid the fat contains.

Saturated fat can raise your LDL or bad cholesterol. This is found in these dairy products: butter, cheese, whole milk, ice cream, and cream. This can also be found in fatty meats.

Vegetable oils that are solid at room temperature, such as coconut oil, palm oil, and palm kernel oil, are also saturated fats.

Unsaturated fats can help lower LDL cholesterol levels. There are two kinds: mono-unsaturated fats and polyunsaturated fats. Mono-saturated fats include olive oil and canola oil, while polyunsaturated fats include sunflower, corn, and safflower.

Some oils that are considered to have excellent health benefits are a combination: flaxseed (linseed) oil has 18% monounsaturated fat, 75% polyunsaturated fat, and 7% saturated fat, whereas hemp seed oil has 15% monounsaturated fat, 75% polyunsaturated fat, and 10% saturated fat.

Another type of fat, known as trans fats, is created when vegetable oil is hardened in a process called hydrogenation, which gives it a longer shelf life. These have been shown to be carcinogenic and should be kept out of your diet. Margarine contains hydrogenated fat and should be avoided. It is healthier to eat butter in small quantities rather than margarine. Read food labels to check for hydrogenated fats.

Olive oil is the best for cooking. Try to buy cold pressed organic oils to eat as dressings. Flaxseed oil is good for your health, as is hemp seed oil. Try to avoid frying food if you can, and never use oil that has been heated twice. Oil should be stored in a cool, dark place and used within three months of opening.

Avocados and nuts are good sources of natural beneficial oils.

Carbohydrate

As we saw briefly in chapter one, carbohydrates are found in foods, such as rice, pasta, bread, potatoes, legumes, pulses, grains, and cereals. It seems quite bizarre to me that the healthy whole meal, whole grain, unprocessed versions that are as nature intended are more expensive than those that have been sent through a variety of goodness stripping processes in a factory – processes that render them with low nutritional value.

The keyword you want when choosing the right carbohydrates to eat is "whole." It really means that the product still contains all the goodness nature gave it to begin with. The main reason these foods are so highly processed is convenience. Whole grain products, such as rice and pasta, take longer to cook than their processed counterparts. This is due to the fiber they contain, which takes time to become soft. The health benefits of eating whole grain products more than make up for this small inconvenience. Not only are they still packed full of all the good micronutrients and dietary fiber, but they also taste better, release energy slowly, and keep you feeling full for a lot longer.

It's time to move over unhealthy, processed carbohydrates. Come on in, healthy and tasty whole grains.

By choosing organic whole grains, you really can't do better for your body. Mother Nature always did know best.

Potatoes. There are pros and cons surrounding potatoes. The humble potato is capable of keeping you alive even if it's all you eat – for a while at least. However, it is a starchy carbohydrate, which you want to limit. To make them more valuable to the diet, you can use potatoes without removing their skins. If boiled and left to cool, they accumulate high levels of resistant starch, which is very beneficial to good gut health, providing a food source for healthy gut bacteria. If you love potatoes for their excellent versatility but want to reduce the amount of starch carbohydrate, you can replace them with sweet potatoes instead. Sweet potatoes have many benefits and can reduce sugar cravings.

Protein

Meat, fish, legumes, whole grains, seeds, nuts, and eggs all contain protein.

Red meat, beef, lamb, and pork all contain saturated fat that can increase unhealthy cholesterol levels. They also contain an enzyme that has been linked to certain types of cancer and diabetes. Processed red meat, such as bacon, sausages, ham, hotdogs, and so on, is doubly bad because their processing increases the carcinogens they contain. For these reasons, their consumption should be limited.

Lean white meat, such as turkey, chicken, or rabbit, is a healthier option to include in your diet.

Fish, particularly oily fish, such as salmon, is a great option as it contains high levels of Omega-3 oils that benefit heart health.

However, you don't require animal protein at all and can get a sufficient amount from other vegetable sources.

Vitamins

Fat-soluble vitamins A, D, and E are needed for healthy bones and teeth, healthy skin, tissue repair, and disease prevention. Vitamin K is used for energy production, fighting infection, blood clotting, and healthy bones.

Water-soluble vitamins B and C are needed for energy production using fat and protein, cell growth, nervous system, red blood cell production, fighting infection, healing wounds, and as an antioxidant to prevent cell damage.

Vitamins can be obtained by eating plenty of high-quality, nutrient-rich fruits and vegetables, lean meat, and fish.

Minerals

Iron, calcium, zinc, iodine, magnesium, selenium, phosphorus, and potassium are the main minerals you need. Trace minerals include fluorine, copper, cobalt, chromium, manganese, and molybdenum. These are needed for red blood cell production, strong teeth, bones, and muscles, hormonal balance, blood clotting, strong immune system, wound healing, healthy thyroid function, nerve and muscle function, and blood pressure.

Eat a good variety of vegetables, particularly leafy green vegetables, fruits, whole grains, seeds, pulses, nuts, shellfish, and lean meat.

Fiber

This is essential for healthy bowel function. It helps lower cholesterol. It also regulates appetite and helps control hunger.

Fiber can be found in whole grains, pulses, lentils, fruits, vegetables, nuts, and seeds.

Chapter 3

Getting the Right Balance

We are going to talk a little about energy production. Your body's preferred energy source is glucose. Glucose is the form of sugar your body obtains from the food you eat. Some foods, such as simple starchy carbohydrates that include processed white bread, pasta, rice, cakes, biscuits, and so on, can provide us with high levels of glucose.

The problem with this is that although your body likes glucose to provide instant energy, any glucose your body does not use cannot be left in your bloodstream for long. This is because having a high blood sugar level is very bad for your health. It can lead to illnesses, such as heart disease, cancer, and diabetes.

When you flood your body with glucose after eating sugary or simple carbohydrate foods, it produces insulin. The insulin goes around your body, telling the cells that there is glucose available for energy. Some of the glucose that isn't used is taken to your liver and lean muscle, where it is stored as glycogen, ready for later use. If there is still too much glucose in the body, it will be converted to fat. If you continue to eat excess sugar and simple carbs, you will gain ever-increasing amounts of fat.

Even more worrying is the more glucose that remains in your bloodstream, as your body releases more insulin to cope with it. When your body's cells are being constantly bombarded by the insulin, telling them to use the glucose for energy (that the cells don't need), the cells start ignoring the insulin. This causes the body to produce even more insulin in response, as it has to get the glucose out of the bloodstream. It's a vicious cycle.

When this occurs, it is called insulin resistance, and it is exceedingly common. If you have belly fat around your middle, the likelihood is that you are already insulin resistant. Here is the bit you really need to know: ***insulin resistance is a precursor to diabetes***. It's a warning sign; it means it's time to take action.

Excess insulin also promotes the release of the stress hormone cortisol. Cortisol sets up an inflammation response in your body and, over time, can cause long-term pain and discomfort in your joints and muscles.

When you go on a diet, you typically eat fewer calories. This stimulates your body to use the glycogen stored in your liver and lean muscle tissue. It is kept in a water base, so the initial weight you lose is simply the loss of that fluid as the glycogen is used up. No fat was turned into energy to achieve this.

Your metabolism is supposed to use glucose to produce energy to run your body and fuel your brain and muscles if you need to carry out physical activity. It also provides energy to your muscles to keep you warm.

However, when your body runs out of glucose to do these things, it has to turn to your secondary energy source – fat. When you run out of energy-rich glucose, your body breaks down the fat in your fat cells and uses that for energy instead. When you're dieting, this is what you want. You want your body to use your stored fat for energy. Therefore, you need to provide it with less readily available glucose.

You need to redress the balance and retune your body, not by starving it of carbohydrates but by providing the right type of carbohydrates in the right proportion to proteins and fats in the form of whole grains. Essential fatty acids are crucial in helping move stored fats out of the fat cells (adipose tissue) so they can be used for energy.

Chapter 4

How to Meal Plan

1. First, set aside a time once a week to decide on your meal plan for the week. Make sure you won't be disturbed, and gather all the things you will need to make meal planning as simple as possible. These things are:
   - Pen and paper
   - Your schedule for the coming week
   - Your favorite recipe books or websites

2. Next, look at your schedule, and note any days when you will need to make food in advance. You may choose to cook some meals in advance anyway, just for convenience and so you don't need to cook every day.

3. Think about the meals you really enjoy eating. If you like takeout, then rather than buying it, you can make your own healthy version at home. Find recipes online, or use cookbooks you have. I certainly have my favorite websites and cookbooks to find recipes; I'm sure you do, too.

4. There are a few tricks you can incorporate, such as cooking a large batch of something to make into several different meals. Bolognese sauce is a great example.

You can turn it into a whole range of different meals: spaghetti Bolognese, cottage pie, lasagna, baked potato filling, chili con carne, stuffed vegetables, fajitas, tacos, or burritos – in fact, anything you can think of. So rather than make a small amount, make a large batch, and freeze it in smaller containers for use at your convenience. Don't only do this with Bolognese; do it with other meals, too. Think of how you can make batches of food if you have a large enough freezer. If you roast a chicken, don't just use the meat; boil up the bones, and make a chicken broth. This is great to use in stocks to add flavor to other dishes, along with lots of nutrients.

Don't forget that if you want to reduce carbs, you can replace pasta, such as spaghetti, with "spiralized" vegetables, or replace pasta sheets with slices of vegetables. I like using zucchini instead of spaghetti and zucchini or sweet potato as lasagna sheets. You can also use spaghetti squash to replace spaghetti or make cauliflower rice with your food processor. Just try to think outside the box, and be creative. Meal planning is a wonderful way to help you do this.

5. Calculate how many meals you will need for the week. Don't forget to include snacks and drinks, too.

6. Decide how to keep your meal plan. Are you going to print off a template to fill out by hand so you can stick it on your fridge for everyone to see? Or would you prefer to keep it on your computer? I personally find a bit of a

blend works best, and I fill out a template on my computer and then print it off. It shows each day of the week along the top of the sheet, with the meals for the day and snacks in between below each day.

7. Now, use a blank piece of paper, and do three brainstorming sessions (you can use your recipe books and online resources to help you here). First, write down a bunch of different breakfast options; things like smoothies, porridge oats with berries, and poached egg with spinach and mushrooms are all quick healthy and nutritious.

   Next, think about lunch. Think about easy, healthy meals that you can take to work and on the go. Be creative, and make the food varied, interesting, and filling. You can eat as much veg as you like with minimal effect on your blood sugar or your waistline. The fiber in veggies also keeps you feeling full and is great for gut health. So, fill up on those veggies!

   Next, it's the supper menu. Go for great flavor, color, and visual appeal here, as well as speed and ease of preparation. Once you have a whole load of ideas (more than you require), get your meal plan chart, and mark on it the days when meals require preparation in advance because of family activities.

8. Now, using the proportion model (carbohydrates, proteins, vegetables, etc.) that you learned about earlier, plan out meals using your brainstorming sheets for each day. Try to keep the menu well balanced. Remember, if there are a lot of carbs eaten at breakfast,

you can reduce the amount at a later meal; just try to keep each day as balanced as you can.

Remember that weight should be lost gradually. To achieve the best results, reduce your calorie intake a little each week until you eat the recommended daily amount for your needs. By doing things gradually, you are more likely to succeed.

With meal planning, variety is the spice of life. You may have to change things up a few times before you're happy with your final plan.

9. When you've completed your meal plan for the week, write out your shopping list to go with it. Check to see what you already have in stock so you don't double up on the ingredients. You may find this tricky to begin with, but before long, you'll be an expert.

As you gain confidence, your expertise will grow, and you'll be able to write up your weekly meal plans in no time at all. Take note of any particularly successful meals so that you can use them again. Don't forget to include some healthy snacks and treats, such as fresh fruit, nuts, and seeds. Even the occasional piece of dark chocolate can stimulate metabolism and aid weight loss.

Conclusion

In conclusion, I hope that you can see how effective meal planning can be, not only as an aid to weight loss but also as an aid to a happier, healthier life – free from the stress and strain of continually wondering what you're going to eat next.

If you can do meal planning and shop only for the foods on your plan, then you will very quickly start seeing results, not only in terms of your waistline (thanking you for cutting all the sugary garbage out of your diet) but also in terms of your health, bank balance, and food anxiety levels. You will be delighted to have such a wonderful, healthy range of great-tasting, nutrient-packed meals. You will feel the benefits, too, from more energy, better sleep, improved health, and a happier and more relaxed you.

It can be challenging to get into the habit of making these meal plans, but please persevere. Only you can make it happen, and I can assure you that it is totally worth it!

And remember to share how well these meal planning and organization tips work for you. You can do that by writing a review in your Amazon account under Your Orders > Digital Orders.

Thank you,

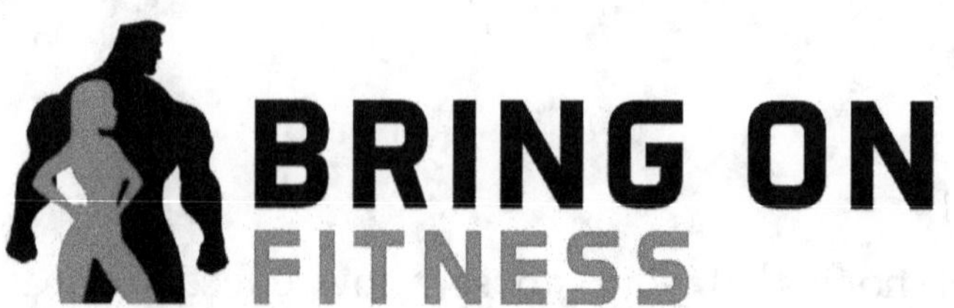

References

Alimentarium.org

Healthline.com

Low GI Cookbook by Louise Blair

So What do you Eat? By Liz Cook

The Food Doctor "Healing Foods for Mind and Body" by Vicki Edgson & Ian Marber

Zest for Life by Conner Middelmann-Whitney